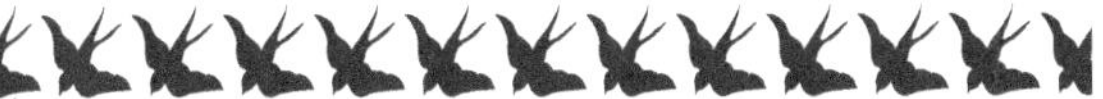

KIDNEY INFECTION TREATMENT

KIDNEY SUPPORTING RECOVERY AT HOME: NATURAL REMEDIES AND LIFESTYLE CHANGES FOR KIDNEY HEALTH

DR. ESTHER J. RAMAGE

ABOUT THE AUTHOR

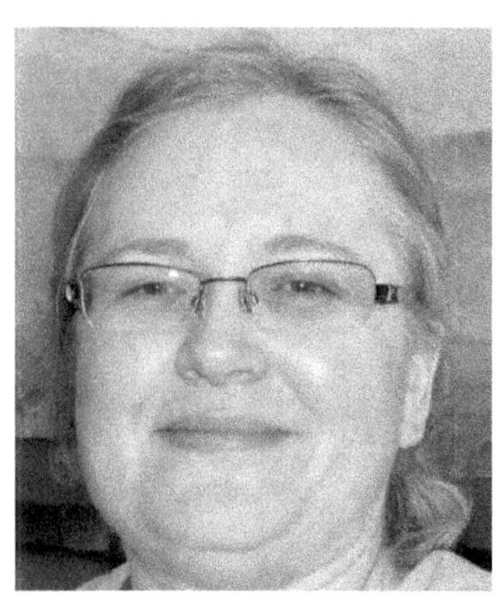 Dr. Esther J. Ramage is a renowned nutritionist, chef, and author who graduated from Harvard University's esteemed Nutritional Science program. Dr. Ramage, with her special knowledge of scientific nutrition as well as culinary arts, is committed to enabling people to live mindfully and use natural solutions to reach their ideal health.

Drawing from her wealth of knowledge and years of experience, Dr. Ramage offers readers a transforming path to kidney health in Kidney Supporting Recovery at Home: Natural Remedies and Lifestyle Changes for Kidney Health. Her engaging, straightforward writing style empowers readers to take charge of their health by making difficult health ideas understandable and doable.

Due to her love for natural medicine, Dr. Ramage has gained recognition as a prominent expert in holistic health from audiences all over the globe. Whether via her books, seminars, or one-on-one conversations, Dr. Ramage never stops encouraging and advising people as they pursue robust health. Accept her expertise and learn how effective lifestyle modifications and natural therapies can be for improving the health of your kidneys and general vigor.

REPRODUCTION RIGHTS

Warning

This book's content is meant purely for educational purposes; it is not meant to be medical advice. Before making any modifications to your food, way of life, or fitness routine, get medical advice. Any losses or unfavorable effects resulting from using the material in this book are not the responsibility of the author or publisher.

TABLE OF CONTENTS

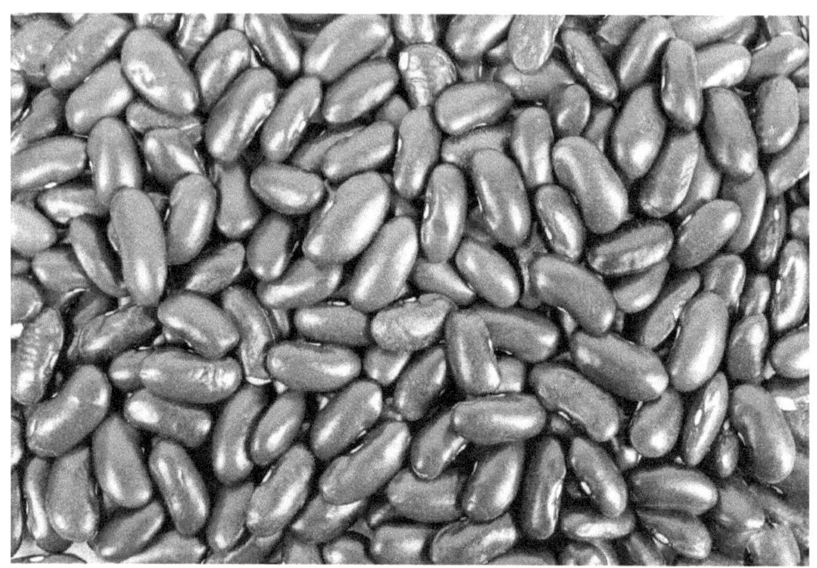

Kidney Beans

INTRODUCTION TO KIDNEY INFECTIONS

OVERVIEW OF KIDNEY FUNCTION AND THEIR VITAL ROLE IN THE BODY

The two bean-shaped organs that make up the kidneys are situated under the rib cage, on each side of the spine. They filter blood, eliminate waste, extra fluid, and electrolytes through the urine they produce, all of which are vital to the body's general health. In addition, the kidneys are essential for maintaining pH balance, controlling blood pressure, and generating hormones like erythropoietin, which promotes the creation of red blood cells. They also aid in the activation of vitamin D, which is essential for healthy bones.

Maintaining homeostasis depends on the kidneys operating properly, and any interference, such as an infection, may cause serious health problems.

AREA OF RISK AND FREQUENCY CAUSES OF KIDNEY INFECTIONS

Bacteria, most commonly Escherichia coli (E. coli), often cause pyelonephritis, the medical term for kidney infections, when they travel up from the lower urinary system to the kidneys. Nevertheless, infections that travel via the bloodstream might also cause them to form. Urinary tract infections (UTIs) that go untreated or come back often, urinary tract anatomical abnormalities, kidney stones, and diseases that restrict urine flow are among the main reasons.

There are many different illnesses and lifestyle choices that might increase the risk of kidney infections. Because of their shorter urethras, which provide germs with better access to the bladder and kidneys, women are more likely to have these infections.

Additional risk variables consist of:

Blockages in the Urinary Tract: Kidney stones, an enlarged prostate, or congenital anomalies may block the flow of urine, which provides an ideal environment for germs to grow.

Weakened Immune System: The body's capacity to fight infections might be hampered by diseases like diabetes, HIV/AIDS, or the use of immunosuppressive medications.

Vesicoureteral reflux (VUR): a disorder that increases the risk of infection by causing urine to flow backward from the bladder to the kidneys. Regular Catheter Use: Using a catheter on a long-term basis may cause infections by introducing germs into the urinary system.

Pregnancy: During pregnancy, there is an increased risk of infection due to hormonal changes and strain on the urinary system.

KIDNEY INFECTION SYMPTOMS AND EARLY WARNING INDICATORS

Early detection of kidney infection symptoms is essential for effective treatment and avoiding life-threatening consequences like sepsis or kidney damage. The severity of the symptoms might vary; however, they usually consist of: **Persistent ache:** A dull, agonizing ache that may spread to the belly or groin, located in the lower back or on either side (flank pain).

High temperature and chills: These symptoms, which are often accompanied by sweating and chills, are the body's reaction to an infection.

Nausea and Vomiting: The body's reaction to the infection often results in digestive problems. Urinary Symptoms: murky, foul-smelling, or bloody urine; increased frequency of urination; an urgent desire to pee; and painful urination (dysuria).

Fatigue and Weakness: As the infection progresses, general malaise and an overall sense of being poorly are common. **Confusion:** A severe kidney infection may manifest as confusion or impaired mental state, particularly in older individuals.

To stop the infection from becoming worse, early action is essential. It's critical to get medical help right away if you have any of these symptoms, particularly if they are accompanied by a fever and excruciating pain.

CHAPTER 1

THE ROLE OF NATURAL REMEDIES IN KIDNEY INFECTION RECOVERY

The supplementary function of herbal remedies in conjunction with medical care Natural treatments may aid in the healing process, even if medical intervention—mainly antibiotics—is necessary for kidney infections to be adequately treated. While these therapies cannot replace expert medical care, they may support traditional medical treatments by reducing symptoms, strengthening the immune system, and enhancing kidney function in general. Including natural therapies in your recuperation plan might ease pain, hasten healing, and possibly stop infections in the future. To prevent any possible interactions, it is essential to speak with a healthcare professional prior to beginning any natural therapy, particularly if you are also on prescribed drugs.

Hydration is the cornerstone of healthy kidneys.

One of the most crucial natural methods for healing from a kidney infection is staying well hydrated. Drinking plenty of water supports the body's natural detoxifying processes by removing germs from the urinary system, lowering the amount of bacteria in the kidneys. Maintaining enough hydration reduces the likelihood of germs growing in urine and lessens the pain caused by urinating while sick. If your doctor advises it, try to drink 8 to 10 glasses of water a day, or more, to maintain the best possible health of your urinary system.

Herbal Treatments: Reducing Inflammation and Promoting Healing
Traditional medicine has used a few plants to promote kidney health and reduce infection symptoms.

Cranberry: It's generally known that cranberry juice or supplements may stop germs from sticking to the walls of the urinary system, which makes it more difficult for infections to start or worsen. Frequent ingestion may help avoid kidney infections and speed up the healing process thereafter.

Parsley: Because of its diuretic properties, parsley

may help boost urine output and clear the kidneys of germs. It may be drunk as a tea or mixed with food.

Marshmallow Root: Known for its calming qualities, marshmallow root helps lessen urinary tract irritation, relieving the pain brought on by kidney infections.

Horsetail: This plant has long been used as an anti-inflammatory and diuretic, encouraging the flow of urine while easing discomfort and swelling.

You may take these herbal medicines as teas, extracts, or supplements, but it's best to speak with a healthcare professional to be sure they're suitable for your particular situation.

Probiotics: Stabilizing the Microbiota to

Enhance Renal Function

Probiotics, beneficial bacteria that maintain a balanced gut flora, may help the healing process after kidney infections. The immune system and the gut microbiome are intimately related, and a healthy microbiome may help stop the proliferation of pathogenic bacteria that might lead to illnesses. Probiotics have the potential to mitigate the adverse effects of antibiotics, including diarrhea, by reestablishing the normal balance of bacteria in the gastrointestinal tract. Probiotic-rich diets include fermented foods like sauerkraut, kefir, yogurt, and others; they may also be taken as supplements.

Apple Cider Vinegar: An Organic Antimicrobial Because of its antibacterial qualities, apple cider vinegar is a well-liked natural therapy that may help fight kidney infection-causing germs. It is thought to provide an alkaline environment in the body, which deters dangerous germs from growing there. Furthermore, acetic acid, which is included in apple cider vinegar, aids in the removal of toxins from the body. Typically, you would combine one or two teaspoons of apple cider vinegar with a glass of water and drink it every day. It should, however, be taken with caution, particularly in those who already have renal problems or are taking drugs that might impair kidney function.

Garlic is an all-natural immune system and antibiotic. For generations, people have used garlic as a natural antibacterial and immune system strengthener. Allicin, one of its constituents, has strong antiviral, antifungal, and antibacterial qualities. Garlic may boost immunity and ward off infection when included in a diet throughout kidney illness recuperation. Fresh garlic is the most powerful form; however, if fresh garlic is intolerable, garlic pills may still be helpful.

Diet is critical for recovering from kidney infection.

Supporting the body's recuperation after a kidney infection is mostly dependent on eating a diet high in nutrients. Pay attention to eating things that are easy on the kidneys and may lower inflammation, like:

Leafy greens: packed with vitamins and antioxidants that boost the immune system and lower inflammation.

Berries: Rich in antioxidants and possessing anti-inflammatory qualities, blueberries, strawberries, and raspberries may help promote healing.

Whole Grains: These kidney-friendly foods, which include quinoa, brown rice, and oats, deliver you steady energy.

Healthy Fats: Essential fatty acids from avocados, almonds, seeds, and olive oil boost immunological function and cellular repair.

Reducing salt consumption is also critical to avoid fluid retention, which may worsen kidney infection symptoms and lessen the strain on the kidneys.

Perks Of Combining Medical Treatment With Natural Remedies

Enhanced Relieving of Symptoms For more thorough symptom relief, natural therapies combined with traditional medical treatments might be helpful. While natural therapies may help reduce related symptoms, including pain, irritation, and inflammation, medicines are necessary to eradicate the infection. Herbal teas and calming foods, for instance, may alleviate discomfort in the urinary system, while dietary changes and increased hydration can lessen symptoms like flank pain and frequent urination.

Immune function support

Probiotics, garlic, and certain vitamins are examples of natural therapies that may strengthen immune system function and make it easier for the body to fight against infections. A robust immune response depends on a balanced population of gut bacteria; which probiotics may help restore. Antibiotics work in tandem with garlic's antibacterial qualities to strengthen the body's fight against microorganisms.

Reduced negative reactions
Side effects from antibiotics and other medical treatments include weariness, altered gut flora, and gastrointestinal disorders. Natural treatments that improve gut health and lower inflammation, such as probiotics and ginger, may lessen these adverse effects. For example, probiotics may help prevent diarrhea brought on by antibiotics, while ginger can aid with nausea and an upset stomach.

Assistance with Renal Health and Function Overall kidney health may be supported by natural therapies like apple cider vinegar, enough water, and dietary changes. Maintaining enough hydration eases the load on the kidneys by removing germs and toxins. Kidney function may be supported by the alkaline environment that apple cider vinegar helps to maintain. Dietary adjustments that boost kidney function and help ward against infections in the future include cutting down on salt and eating more foods that are beneficial for the kidneys.

Encouragement of Quicker Recovery Natural therapies may hasten healing by enhancing general wellbeing and assisting the body's healing processes, natural therapies may hasten the healing process. For instance, anti-inflammatory foods and herbs help lessen inflammation and swelling, resulting in symptom alleviation more quickly. A balanced diet and enough water may boost energy levels and assist the body's healing processes, hastening the body's recuperation.

Recurrence Prevention

Kidney infections may be avoided in the future by including natural therapies in a thorough treatment program. Cranberry supplements, for example, have been shown to have a role in lowering the risk of recurring infections by inhibiting bacteria's ability to adhere to the urinary tract. Modifications to diet and lifestyle, such as increased water intake, may also support urinary tract health and lower the risk of recurring infections.

A holistic approach to health is promoted by combining medical care with natural therapies, which not only address the current illness but also promote general well-being. This method takes a more holistic approach to fostering balance and health by taking into account the body's linked systems. Through the management of fundamental elements including immune system performance, dietary patterns, and way of life decisions, people may improve their health and quality of life.

Patients may take an active role in their own rehabilitation when medical therapies are combined with natural cures. Awareness and use of complementary therapies increase patients' compliance with treatment and health responsibility. This involvement can lead to better symptom management, a greater sense of control over one's health, and better adherence to medical treatments.

Carefulness When Using Home Medication

Seek advice from medical professionals. It is important to speak with a healthcare professional before beginning any home remedy, particularly if you are receiving medical treatment at the moment or have underlying medical concerns. Certain treatments may worsen pre-existing problems or interfere with prescription drugs. A medical expert can advise you on the suitability and safety of certain treatments, depending on your unique medical requirements.

Don't rely solely on home remedies.

Although they have their advantages, home cures shouldn't take the place of professional medical care. To successfully eradicate kidney infections, antibiotics or other specified therapies are necessary for kidney infections in order to successfully eradicate the infection. Using just natural treatments in place of proper medical care may exacerbate an illness, cause complications, or result in long-term problems. Home remedies should be used in addition to medical treatment, not as a replacement.

Recognize any potential sensitivities or allergies Herbs, vitamins, and certain foods are examples of natural therapies that may trigger allergic responses or sensitivities in some people. To be sure you don't have a negative response, do a patch test or speak with your doctor before taking a new treatment. Keep an eye out for any allergy symptoms, such as rash, itching, or upset stomach.

Apply the remedy at the suggested doses. For all at-home medicines, including essential oils and herbal supplements, abide by the suggested doses and directions. Overuse or improper dosing may cause toxic consequences or adverse effects. For example, consuming too much apple cider vinegar might harm tooth enamel or induce gastrointestinal distress. Always follow the instructions, and if you have any questions regarding dosing, speak with a healthcare professional.

Take into account potential drug interactions. Prescription drugs and many natural treatments may interact negatively, changing the prescription drug's efficacy or producing negative side effects. Herbal supplements, such as garlic, have the potential to impact blood coagulation and interfere with anticoagulant drugs. Inform your doctor of any over-the-counter drugs you take to avoid drug interactions.

Keep an eye out for side effects. After starting a home cure, pay attention to any side effects or changes to your health. Headaches, skin rashes, and stomach problems are common adverse effects. Should you encounter any atypical or severe symptoms, stop using the medication immediately and see a doctor? Make Use of Reputable, High-Quality Products Purchase essential oils or herbal supplements from reputable vendors to ensure they are pure and uncontaminated. It's critical to choose supplements that have undergone effectiveness and purity testing since some supplements may be contaminated or contain dangerous chemicals.

Continue using a balanced approach. Combine natural healing methods with a well-rounded regimen that includes enough sleep, healthy food, and enough water. It may not be the best idea to rely solely on treatments and ignore other aspects of health. The greatest results may be obtained via a comprehensive strategy that incorporates natural therapies, medical care, and lifestyle modifications.

Steer clear of dangerous or unproven remedies. Remedies that don't have scientific backing or might be dangerous should be avoided. Certain over-the-counter treatments for kidney infections may be hazardous or lack scientific backing. Steer clear of unproven therapies, and trust only treatments with strong evidence supporting them or those that medical experts suggest.

Stay current and informed. Over time, studies on natural cures and health advice may change. Keep up with the most recent research findings and recommendations on kidney infections and over-the-counter treatments. Consult medical professionals on a regular basis to make sure your treatment plan is still safe and efficient.

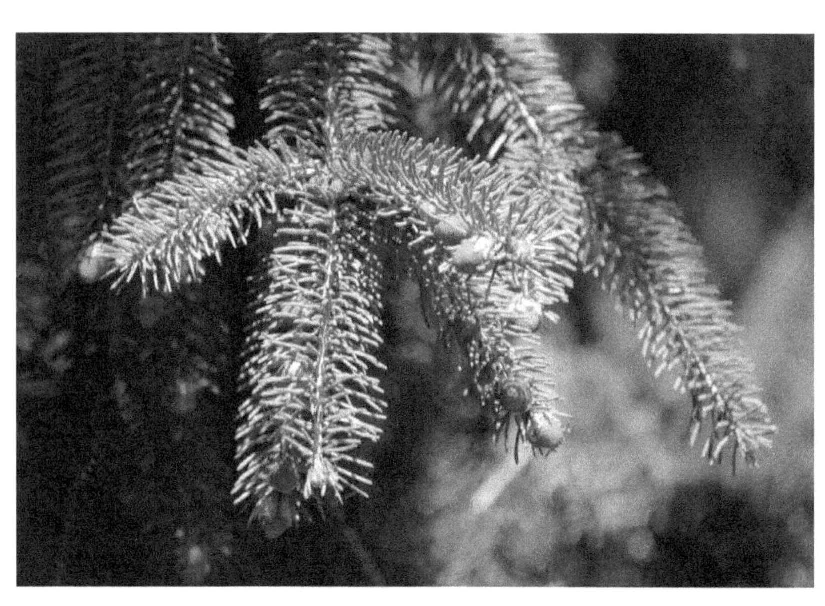

CHAPTER 2

TOP HOME REMEDIES FOR KIDNEY INFECTION RECOVERY

Pyelonephritis, another name for kidney infections, is a dangerous condition that has to be treated by a doctor. Nonetheless, in addition to medical care, certain natural therapies may aid in healing and reduce symptoms. Prior to attempting any new treatments, always get medical advice, particularly if you have a kidney infection. The following natural therapies might be beneficial:

Drink plenty of water

- Importance: Getting enough water enhances kidney function and aids in the removal of microorganisms from the urinary system.

- Suggested Drinking: Try to have 8–10 glasses of water each day. Herbal drinks, including ginger or chamomile, provide additional advantages.

Juice from Cranberries

- Significance: Compounds in cranberry juice may help keep germs from adhering to the urinary system.

- Select unsweetened 100% cranberry juice. Have a little glass every day to promote healthy urinary function.

Onion

- The inherent antibacterial qualities of garlic may aid in the defense against illnesses.

- Suggestion: Include fresh garlic in your meals. Garlic supplements are also an option, but check with your doctor about the right amount.

Ginger

- Ginger's antibacterial and anti-inflammatory qualities may aid in the body's healing process.

- Suggested Use: Incorporate fresh ginger into your dishes or sip ginger tea. After speaking with your doctor, you may also take supplements containing raw ginger or eat it raw.

Tea with Dandelion

- The diuretic qualities of dandelion root aid in boosting urine production and may promote renal health.

- Prepare dandelion tea per the directions on the box and sip one to two cups per day. Consult your healthcare practitioner to be sure it is suitable for your situation.

Vinegar made from apples

- The antimicrobial qualities of apple cider vinegar may aid in maintaining the right pH balance in the urinary system.

- Combine a glass of water with 1-2 teaspoons of apple cider vinegar. Consume this blend once or twice day. If you are sensitive to stomach acid, use this cure with caution.

Supplemental Nutrition

- Probiotics may help avoid recurring urinary tract infections and maintain gut health.

- Incorporate foods high in probiotics, such as fermented vegetables, kefir, and yogurt, into your diet. Probiotic supplements may also be helpful; choose a reputable brand and speak with your doctor.

Repose and Calm

- Your body needs enough sleep in order to efficiently fight off infections and heal.

- Make sure you receive enough rest and steer clear of physically demanding activities. Establishing a tranquil, soothing space might also help with your general recuperation.

Steer clear of irritants

- Specific meals and beverages may aggravate symptoms by irritating the urinary system.

- While recuperating, minimize or stay away from coffee, alcohol, hot, and acidic meals.

CHAPTER 3.

LIFESTYLE CHANGES TO SUPPORT KIDNEY HEALTH

Maintain Hydration: The key to good kidney function

Staying well hydrated is essential to preserving renal health. Water aids the kidneys' ability to remove waste from the blood and excrete it in urine. Getting enough water lowers the risk of kidney stones and urinary tract infections, which may result in kidney infections. It also dilutes urine. Try to get in at least 8 to 10 glasses of water a day, or more if your doctor suggests it. That being said, people with certain renal problems may need to closely monitor their fluid intake, so it's crucial to customize your hydration to meet your unique requirements.

Adopt a Kidney-Friendly Diet.

A nutrient-rich, well-balanced diet promotes kidney health in general and aids in the treatment of pre-existing renal disorders.

Important dietary adjustments consist of: Reduce Sodium Consumption: Over soiling with salt may raise blood pressure, straining the kidneys and making renal disease worse. Eliminate salt from your diet by sticking to fresh, whole foods, using herbs and spices in place of salt, and avoiding processed foods.

Consume Phosphorus and Potassium Moderately: Controlling the amount of potassium and phosphorus consumed is crucial for renal disease patients to prevent problems. Because foods rich in these minerals include potatoes, bananas, oranges, and dairy products, it's important to follow your healthcare practitioner's dietary recommendations.

Incorporate foods high in antioxidants: Leafy greens, berries, and other antioxidant-rich fruits and vegetables aid in reducing inflammation and promoting healthy kidney function. Oxidative stress, which over time may harm kidney cells, is fought by antioxidants.

Pay Attention to Lean Proteins: Consuming too much protein may strain the kidneys, especially in those with impaired renal function. Choose plant-based sources of protein, such as beans and lentils, and lean proteins, such as fish and poultry. Modify your protein consumption in accordance with medical advice.

Continue to eat healthily.

It's critical for kidney health to reach and maintain a healthy weight. Being obese raises the chance of getting diseases like diabetes and hypertension, which are major contributors to kidney damage. The keys to managing weight are a balanced diet and regular exercise. Try to get at least 150 minutes a week of moderate activity, such as cycling, swimming, or walking, to help you maintain your weight and improve your cardiovascular health.

Control blood sugar and blood pressure. Diabetes and high blood pressure are two main risk factors for renal disease. To preserve kidney health, these disorders must be regularly monitored and managed. Blood pressure may be controlled by making lifestyle adjustments such as eating a balanced diet, exercising often, and consuming less sodium. To avoid kidney damage, diabetics must maintain stable blood sugar levels through food, exercise, and taking their medications as directed.

Give Up Smoking and Drink Less Alcohol Kidney health may be adversely affected by smoking and binge drinking. Smoking damages the kidneys' ability to filter blood, lowers blood flow to them, and raises the risk of kidney disease. Both general health and renal health may be improved by quitting smoking. In a similar vein, consuming too much alcohol may harm the liver, cause dehydration, raise blood pressure, and severely impact the kidneys. If you decide to use alcohol, be sure you do it responsibly and in accordance with suggested dosages.

Maintain proper hygiene to avoid infections. Kidney health depends on preventing infections, especially urinary tract infections (UTIs). If neglected, UTIs may result in kidney infections. UTIs may be avoided by following basic hygiene practices, such as drinking plenty of water, peeing after sexual activity, and wiping after using the restroom from front to back. Kidney problems may also be decreased by rapidly treating any infections and following up with medical professionals.

Managing Stress and Sleep: The Importance of Rest for Healing Sleep's healing properties The body's capacity to mend and rejuvenate depends heavily on sleep, which is a basic element of both recuperation and general health. The body goes through vital functions that promote immune function, tissue repair, and detoxification while you sleep deeply. These functions are crucial for kidney health and infection recovery. Getting enough sleep lowers blood pressure, eases inflammation, and supports the hormonal balance that affects kidney function. Getting seven to nine hours of adequate sleep every night is essential for kidney infection recovery because it helps the body concentrate on repair and restoration.

Stress and How It Affects Kidney Function Prolonged stress may worsen kidney disease by raising blood pressure and causing the release of stress hormones like cortisol, which can make kidney issues worse. Stress may also contribute to kidney-damaging habits, such as eating poorly, not drinking enough water, and abusing drugs like alcohol and caffeine. Thus, controlling stress is essential for maintaining kidney function and promoting infection recovery. Stress reduction promotes healthy kidneys by lowering blood pressure, reducing inflammation, and enhancing general wellbeing.

Methods of Relaxation to Aid in Healing When included in everyday routines, relaxation methods may greatly reduce stress and aid in healing. Activities that help relax the nervous system, reduce cortisol levels, and enhance the quality of sleep include gradual muscle relaxation, yoga, meditation, and deep breathing exercises.

Regular participation in these activities may improve mental clarity, encourage emotional equilibrium, and aid in the body's healing processes. Walking and mild stretching are additional physical activities that may enhance circulation and reduce stress, both of which are beneficial to kidney health.

Establishing a calm sleep environment

Establishing a relaxing and comfortable sleep environment is critical for maximizing recovery sleep. This entails keeping the bedroom calm, cold, and dark, utilizing cozy bedding, and creating a regular sleep routine. Before going to bed, avoiding devices and mentally taxing activities might help your body recognize when it's time to relax. A calming nighttime practice, like reading a book, stretching lightly, or having a warm bath, may also help the body and mind get ready for sound sleep.

A well-balanced routine's role
Maintaining a healthy balance between work and leisure activities is crucial for stress management and rehabilitation. Overworking oneself or not making time for relaxation a priority may result in burnout, which is detrimental for one's physical and emotional well-being. Making time for hobbies, taking frequent breaks throughout the day, and going outside may all help boost wellbeing and replenish energy. In order to continue healing and preserve kidney health, a well-balanced regimen that includes time for self-care and relaxation is essential.

Looking for help with stress management
Sometimes further assistance is needed to manage

stress. Joining a support group or talking with a counselor or therapist might provide helpful coping mechanisms and emotional support. Speaking with a professional or someone you can trust about worries, difficulties, or stresses may help ease psychological strain and promote a more optimistic attitude towards recovery for people recuperating from a kidney infection.

Mind-Body Harmony and Recovery

Healing is largely influenced by the mind-body link, with emotional and stress management having a direct impact on physical healing. Stress management techniques, positive thinking, and mindfulness may improve the body's capacity for healing by strengthening the immune system and lessening the load of stress-related hormones on the kidneys. Resilience may be increased by practicing thankfulness and maintaining an optimistic outlook, which will make it simpler to handle the difficulties of rehabilitation.

Minimizing Exposure to Dangerous Substances: Preventing Toxins

Recognizing How Toxins Affect Kidney Health The kidneys are crucial organs that remove and filter toxins from the body, but they may become overloaded and harmed by prolonged exposure to toxic chemicals. A number of substances, such as chemicals, pharmaceuticals, food additives, and contaminants in the environment, may damage kidney function and raise the risk of renal disease. It's critical to understand these dangerous compounds and limit exposure to them in order to protect kidney health, particularly while recovering from illnesses.

Reduced Exposure to Pollutants in the Environment

Toxins from the environment, including pesticides, heavy metals, and industrial pollutants, may enter the body via food, water, and the air. These compounds have the potential to build up in the kidneys and cause chronic harm. In order to avoid exposure, choose organic products to lower the amount of pesticides and herbicides that are often used in conventional farming. Reducing pesticide residues may also be achieved by carefully washing fruits and vegetables.

Filter Drinking Water: By eliminating dangerous impurities from tap water, such as lead, chlorine, and other pollutants, a high-quality water filter may lessen the strain on the kidneys. Prevent Being Around Secondhand Smoke: Numerous chemicals included in tobacco smoke may damage the kidneys. You may keep yourself healthier by avoiding places where smoking is permitted and by promoting a smoke-free atmosphere.

Pay Attention to Air Quality: You may lessen the amount of dangerous particles you breathe in that might impair kidney function by minimizing your exposure to outdoor air pollution, such as smog, and by using air purifiers within your home.

Selecting Secure Home Goods Numerous personal care, cosmetic, and home cleaning products include chemicals that may be dangerous to breathe in or absorb through the skin. Phthalates, parabens, and volatile organic compounds (VOCs) are a few examples of these substances that might be harmful to kidney health. In order to reduce exposure: Use eco-friendly or natural cleaning supplies. Choose cleaning solutions with natural components instead of synthetic ones, such as baking soda, vinegar, and essential oils. These products are less likely to contain dangerous chemicals.

Steer clear of synthetic scents: synthetic scents included in many air fresheners, perfumes, and scented goods have the potential to emit dangerous compounds into the atmosphere. Instead, choose for naturally scented or fragrance-free items.

Choose Secure Personal Care Items: Select personal care products that don't include harsh chemicals or artificial additions, such as soaps, lotions, and shampoos. Seek out goods with labels indicating they are non-toxic, organic, or devoid of sulfates and parabens.

Exercise caution when taking supplements and medicines.

Nonsteroidal anti-inflammatory medicines (NSAIDs), over-the-counter painkillers, and certain prescription pharmaceuticals may all be hazardous to the kidneys, particularly if used often or in large quantities. Inadequate use of herbal supplements could be dangerous.

To keep your kidneys safe:

Adhere to Recommended Doses: Never use anything other than as prescribed by your doctor, and refrain from using over-the-counter pharmaceuticals for self-medication. Before beginning a new pharmaceutical regimen, talk to your doctor about any concerns you may have about kidney health.

Refrain from Using NSAIDs Needlessly: NSAIDs may relieve pain and inflammation, but over time, they can also harm the kidneys by decreasing blood supply to them. When feasible, look into other pain treatment methods and use them sparingly.

Look into Herbal Supplementation: Certain herbal supplements have the potential to impair kidney function due to their toxic contents or interactions with medicines. Before taking any supplements, particularly if you already have renal problems, speak with your doctor.

Minimizing Exposure to Dangers at Work Workers in several professions may be exposed to heavy metals, chemicals, and other substances that are harmful to the kidneys. If there is a chance that you may be exposed to such things at work: Use Protective Equipment: To reduce direct contact with hazardous chemicals, use the proper personal protective equipment (PPE), such as gloves, masks, and protective clothes.

Adhere to Safety Instructions: To lower the chance of coming into contact with dangerous substances and materials, follow workplace safety procedures and rules.

Look for routine health monitoring. Regular health examinations and renal function testing may help identify any early indications of kidney impairment if you are exposed to pollutants at work.

Selecting non-toxic substitutes Whenever feasible, use non-toxic substitutes for frequently used items.

As an illustration:

Cookware: Instead of using non-stick pans, which may contain perfluorooctanoic acid (PFOA), a chemical related to kidney damage, choose appliances made of stainless steel, cast iron, or ceramic.

Gardening: Rather of using chemical-based treatments, use natural pest control techniques and fertilizers in your garden. Carpeting and Furniture: Select carpets and furnishings that are devoid of formaldehyde and flame retardants, two substances that may emit toxic vapors.

Acquiring Knowledge about Toxins Making safer decisions may be facilitated by being aware of possible poisons and dangerous materials found in common items.

Do your homework and carefully study labels to avoid components that may be harmful to your kidneys and general health. Being aware of toxins and their effects on the body will enable you to take preventative measures to reduce exposure and protect your kidneys.

CHAPTER 4

MONITORING AND MAINTAINING PROGRESS AT HOME

Monitor health indicators and symptoms continuously.

It's important to monitor your symptoms and general health closely when recuperating from a kidney infection. You may spot such problems early on by keeping a regular eye on important markers, including pain intensity, temperature, urine patterns, and any changes in energy levels.

Keep a daily journal of these symptoms, recording any ameliorations or deteriorations. With this information, your healthcare physician will be able to make educated decisions about your treatment plan during follow-up appointments.

Check the levels of blood sugar and blood pressure. Uncontrolled blood sugar and high blood pressure may aggravate renal problems and make recovery more difficult. It's critical to keep an eye on your blood pressure and glucose levels at home if you have a history of these conditions.

Track and record your data on a regular basis with a dependable blood pressure and blood glucose meter. Supporting kidney health and preventing further complications necessitates maintaining ideal blood pressure and blood sugar levels through medication, dietary adjustments, and lifestyle modifications.

Management of Fluid Intake and Hydration
Kidney function depends on being hydrated, but it's also critical to control fluid consumption based on your unique health requirements. Your healthcare physician can suggest a specific range of fluid consumption based on your situation. Fluid overload or deficiency may cause renal strain. Monitor your daily fluid consumption using a water tracker app or notebook to ensure that you are staying within the prescribed range while still reaching your hydration goals.

Follow the doctor's orders and treatment plans.
For you to heal, you must take your medications as directed. It's important to follow the directions on antibiotics and other prescriptions precisely, even if you feel better before the course is finished.

Antibiotic resistance or the illness may return if dosages are missed or medicine is stopped too soon. You may assist yourself in remembering to take your medications on time by setting reminders or using a pill organizer.

Check your urine frequently, and keep an eye out for changes.

Tests on urine may identify the presence of infection, protein, blood, or other anomalies, which can offer crucial information about kidney health. Use home test strips to keep an eye on your urine for any indications of infection or other problems, as directed by your healthcare practitioner. Changes in the color, smell, or frequency of urine should be noted since these may be early signs of kidney issues. Any unexpected results should be reported right away to your healthcare physician.

Set up and maintain follow-up consultations

Maintaining good kidney healing necessitates regular follow-up sessions with your healthcare provider to assess your recovery.

In order to evaluate your kidney function and general health, your doctor may prescribe blood tests, urine tests, or imaging investigations during these sessions. note any queries or worries you would want to address during these sessions, and don't hesitate to bring up any new problems or symptoms that have emerged since your previous visit.

Continue Eating a Well-Balanced Diet

To aid in healing and stop more kidney damage, a diet that is favorable to the kidneys is essential. As directed by your healthcare practitioner, concentrate on eating a diet high in fruits, vegetables, whole grains, and lean proteins, and limit your consumption of sodium, potassium, and phosphorus. Consider creating a meal plan that is customized to your individual requirements by consulting with a nutritionist. Make sure your diet is in line with your health goals on a regular basis, and alter it as necessary to help you continue to heal.

Participate in regular exercise.

Kidney function may be enhanced by physical exercise via its ability to lower stress, promote general health, and increase circulation. Try some light exercise, like yoga, swimming, or walking;

these might be especially helpful while you're healing. But it's crucial to pay attention to your body and refrain from overdoing it, particularly if you're still feeling discomfort or exhaustion. As your strength recovers, gradually increase your activity level. Before beginning any new fitness program, speak with your healthcare professional.

Continue to learn and understand kidney health.

Gaining knowledge about renal health and the variables that affect it will enable you to play a more active part in your recuperation. Keep up with the most recent findings, available treatments, and lifestyle suggestions for maintaining kidney health. Participating in online support groups, seminars, or reading books may provide insightful information and inspire you to continue with healthy routines.

Ask friends and family for support.

A kidney infection may be difficult to recover from emotionally and physically. Never be afraid to ask for help from friends and family; they may be a source of motivation, assistance with everyday duties, and emotional support. By may maintain your adherence to your rehabilitation plan by updating your loved ones on your progress. Furthermore, think about reaching out to others who have also had kidney infections; peer support may provide insightful comments and guidance.

Assess and modify your schedule as required.

Since recovery is a dynamic process, it's critical to often assess your level of success and modify your regimen as necessary. Don't be afraid to alter tactics or routines if they aren't producing the expected outcomes. Maintaining your success and achieving long-term kidney health will need you to be adaptable and sensitive to your body's demands, whether that means experimenting with new stress-reduction methods, dietary changes, or exercise regimens.

MANAGEING SYMPTOMS AND IDENTIFYING IMPROVEMENTS

Keep a Daily Record of Symptoms A thorough daily symptom record is one of the best tools for monitoring your development and identifying improvements over time. Keep a notebook where you may document any symptoms you have, such as pain intensity, fever, exhaustion, altered urine patterns, and any other pertinent health indicators. Provide specifics, such as the time of day symptoms occur, how severe they are, and any activities or environments that appear to exacerbate or relieve the symptoms. You may use this notebook to monitor changes in your condition and spot trends.

Employ apps for tracking symptoms.
Apps for documenting symptoms digitally might make keeping an eye on your health easier. These applications allow you to frequently record your symptoms, medication use, and other health information. Certain applications may provide reports or graphical representations that facilitate the identification of patterns and advancements over time. Select an app that lets you tailor the monitoring fields to your unique requirements,

and make sure it's simple to use so you'll use it consistently.

Use a pain scale to track your level of pain. Kidney infections often cause pain, so keeping a careful eye on them might provide important information about your prognosis. To assess your pain throughout the day, use a pain scale from 1 to 10, where 1 represents minor discomfort and 10 represents excruciating agony. Note the pain's location, intensity, and kind (sharp, dull, throbbing, etc.). If the frequency and severity of your discomfort decrease over time, improvement should be evident.

Monitor Changes in Urination Patterns Urinary changes are one of the most important markers of kidney health. Keep note of your urine's volume, color, and frequency, as well as any pain or discomfort you have while urinating. Keep an eye out for any bloodstains, discoloration, or strange smells that might indicate an infection or other problems. Possible improvements include a return to regular urine frequency, a clear or light yellow hue, and a lack of pain or discomfort.

Monitor your energy and fatigue levels. Fatigue is often linked to kidney infections and may indicate an infection-related reaction in your body. Every day, score your energy levels on a simple scale of 1 to 5, where 1 represents mild weariness and 5 represents high energy. note any activities that appear to improve your mood or sap your vitality. A good indicator of recovery is an increase in energy, such as feeling more awake, being able to do tasks for longer periods of time, or requiring fewer rest periods.

Be aware of temperature fluctuations and fevers.

A fever is one typical sign of illness. Keep an eye on your body temperature every day, particularly if you've been having fevers. Make sure to take your temperature every day at the same time with a trustworthy thermometer. A decrease in your fever or a return to a normal temperature is a sign that your illness is improving.

Examine your digestive health and appetite

Digestion and appetite might be impacted by kidney illnesses. Keep a food diary and record any changes in your appetite, nausea, or gastrointestinal distress. Gains in this area might include regular digestion, less nausea, and a return to   a   normal   appetite.

Examine your mood and mental clarity.

Confusion, anger, or anxiety may result from infections that affect mood and mental acuity. Every day, monitor your mental health and record any changes in your mood, level of focus, or memory. Enhancements might manifest as improved concentration, emotional stability, and mental clarity—all indicators that your body is healing.

Establish goals and benchmarks.

Establishing precise benchmarks and objectives may aid in more efficient progress measurement. For instance, if pain has been a major problem, establish a goal to get pain under control to a certain number on the pain scale in a predetermined amount of time. You'll be able to see noticeable changes in your condition when you cross these benchmarks.

Talk to your medical professional.

Maintaining regular contact with your healthcare professional is crucial for monitoring your symptoms and identifying any progress. At your follow-up visits, discuss with your physician your symptom diary, tracking information, and any concerns you may have. They may provide you with comfort about your progress, assist you in evaluating the facts, and help you make adjustments to your treatment plan.

Pay attention to your body's signals.

Lastly, pay attention to your body. It's possible that some days feel better than others, and improvement isn't always linear. Be patient with the healing process and pay attention to your body's cues. Even a small but consistent improvement in your symptoms is a good indicator that your self-care and therapy are working.

Knowing When to See a Medical Expert

Prolonged or Getting Worse

It's essential to see a healthcare provider if your symptoms increase over time or if they continue even after you've followed your treatment plan. If after a few days of treatment, the symptoms don't go better, such as persistent or worsening pain, fever, chills, exhaustion, or pain while urinating, there may be consequences or the infection is not responding to treatment. In order to keep the disease from becoming worse, immediate medical intervention   is   required.

Extreme fever or chills

A high temperature (usually greater than 38.3°C, or 101°F) or ongoing chills might indicate that the illness is becoming worse or spreading. It's critical to get medical help right away if you have these symptoms, especially if they are accompanied by shaking or perspiration. A high temperature may indicate a more dangerous illness that has to be treated   right   away,   like   sepsis.

Sharp or severe pain.

An acute or severe discomfort in your belly, sides, or lower back may be a sign of a more serious issue, such as a kidney stone, abscess, or significant infection. This kind of discomfort has to be addressed right away and calls for an appointment with a medical professional. Any sudden or severe pain has to be assessed right away in order to avoid developing other issues.

Urine contains blood.

Having blood in your urine is a sign of a kidney or urinary system problem. Even though some illnesses may cause little quantities of blood to emerge, visible blood or clots should always be examined by a medical practitioner. Urine containing blood may indicate kidney stones, infections, or other severe diseases requiring medical attention.

Loss of appetite, nausea, or vomiting

During a kidney infection, persistent nausea, vomiting, or a substantial appetite loss may be signs that the infection has moved to other regions of your body or is impacting your digestive system. These symptoms may exacerbate your recuperation by causing dehydration. If you have these symptoms, it's important to get in touch with your healthcare provider so that you can decide on the best course of action.

Perplexity or Lack of Direction

Confusion, disorientation, or trouble remaining awake in yourself or someone you are caring for could be indicators of a major consequence, such as sepsis or renal failure. Given that the infection may be impacting the brain or other critical organs, these cognitive abnormalities are warning signs that need to be taken seriously and should be treated right away.

Modifications in Urine

Consultation with a healthcare provider is recommended for significant changes in urine production, such as dark, cloudy, or foul-smelling urine or an inability to pee. These alterations may be a sign of decreasing renal function or urgent problems that need medical attention. Especially the inability to urinate might indicate a serious illness or obstruction that has to be treated right away.

Edema, or swelling

Edema, or swelling in the legs, ankles, feet, or face, may occur if your kidneys aren't working effectively and can't remove extra fluid from your body. It's crucial to see a doctor if you have unusual or prolonged swelling, since this might indicate renal impairment or other significant health problems that need immediate care.

Chest pain or shortness of breath

If the kidneys are failing and fluid accumulates in the lungs (a condition known as pulmonary edema), chest discomfort or shortness of breath may result. These signs may potentially suggest that the infection has progressed to the heart or lungs. Breathing problems or chest discomfort should be handled as a medical emergency, and you should get help right away.

Ongoing Infections

Frequent kidney infections might indicate an underlying illness such as kidney stones, an immune system problem, or an anomaly in the urinary tract's structure. A healthcare provider should conduct a comprehensive investigation into recurrent infections in order to determine the underlying reason and take appropriate action to avoid future infections and possible kidney damage.

After 48–72 hours of treatment, there is no improvement

Usually, after you start antibiotic therapy for a kidney infection, you should feel better in 48 to 72 hours. It's critical to speak with your healthcare physician if symptoms intensify or if you don't see any improvement within this time period. To make sure the infection is successfully treated, they may need to modify your medication, recommend an alternative antibiotic, or order more testing.

Experiencing new or inexplicable symptoms

You should speak with a healthcare provider about any new or unexplained symptoms that appear while you're recovering. Rashes, joint discomfort, or sudden changes in your health might be symptoms of an infection or pharmaceutical side effects. It's crucial that you let your doctor know about them so they can determine if they need to be evaluated separately or have any bearing on your present condition.

Value of Continuous Care and Permanent Child Health

Making Certain of a Full Recovery from Infection After a kidney infection, follow-up treatment is crucial to make sure the infection has completely healed and to avoid any lasting or recurrent problems. Bacteria in the kidneys or urinary system may persist even after symptoms have subsided. Scheduling regular follow-up sessions enables your healthcare practitioner to do the required tests, including blood or urine tests, to verify that the infection has fully healed. By doing this, problems like kidney damage and persistent kidney infections are avoided.

Tracking Kidney Function

Renal function may be impacted by kidney infections, particularly if they are severe or persistent. As part of your follow-up treatment, your kidney function will be monitored by tests such as blood urea nitrogen (BUN) and creatinine levels, which measure how effectively your kidneys are removing waste from your blood. Kidney failure or chronic kidney disease (CKD) may be prevented by promptly intervening when there is a deterioration in kidney function.

Avoiding Repeated Infections

After a kidney infection, a person's chance of getting another infection is higher. The goal of follow-up treatment is to find and treat any underlying conditions, such as kidney stones, abnormalities of the urinary tract, or compromised immune systems, that may be causing recurring infections. To lower the risk of recurring kidney infections, your healthcare professional may recommend preventative treatments such as medication, surgery, or lifestyle modifications.

Prolong Renal Health and Illness Avoidance

Because the kidneys are essential for controlling blood pressure, balancing electrolytes, and filtering waste, maintaining long-term renal health is important for general wellbeing. Follow-up care offers a chance to talk about long-term renal health support methods. This entails controlling kidney disease risk factors through diet, exercise, and medication, such as high blood pressure, diabetes, and obesity. The development of end-stage renal disease or chronic kidney disease may be stopped by early intervention in these areas.

Lifestyle modifications to promote kidney health

A common topic of discussion in follow-up care is lifestyle changes that may support kidney health. These might include dietary advice to limit salt consumption, consume foods that are good for the kidneys, and drink enough water. In addition, your healthcare professional could provide advice on stress reduction, exercise, and avoiding chemicals, drugs, and excessive alcohol intake that might damage the kidneys. By making these adjustments, you may enhance your general quality of life and safeguard your kidneys.

Recognizing and handling issues

Complications from kidney infections might include elevated blood pressure, abscess formation, and kidney scarring. Your healthcare practitioner can identify and successfully treat these issues when you get regular follow-up care. For example, if kidney impairment results in high blood pressure, early intervention may stop the kidneys from becoming worse and lower the risk of cardiovascular disease.

Adherence and Management of Medication

Even after symptoms have subsided, it's crucial to take prescription drugs like antibiotics as directed for the whole duration of the illness if you have a kidney infection. Follow-up care ensures that you understand the importance of medication adherence and offers a chance to discuss any side effects or treatment-related concerns you may have. In addition, your doctor could change your prescription schedule in response to how well you're recovering or the findings of further testing.

Promoting Mental and Emotional Health

It may be difficult to heal from a kidney infection both physically and psychologically. Any mental health issues, such as sadness or anxiety, that may surface during or after recovery are addressed as part of follow-up treatment. In order to assist you in managing the psychological effects of your disease and to enhance your general well-being, your healthcare practitioner may provide you with information, resources, and referrals to counseling services if necessary.

Patient empowerment and education

Attending follow-up visits gives you the opportunity to learn more about your condition and become more involved in maintaining your kidneys over time. Your healthcare provider may give advice on how to spot kidney problems early on, how important it is to have screenings for health issues on a regular basis, and when to get help. Making educated judgments about your health lowers the chance of difficulties in the road and helps you make better decisions about how to care for your kidneys.

Establishing a robust healthcare collaboration

A solid relationship between you and your healthcare provider is fostered by routine follow-up treatment. By maintaining this connection, you may be confident that your healthcare staff is knowledgeable about your medical background, aware of your unique health requirements, and equipped to provide individualized treatment.

Frequent check-ins enable your doctor to monitor your development, modify your treatment plan as necessary, and assist you in preserving the best possible condition of your kidneys.

CHAPTER 5

PREVENTION STRATEGIES TO AVOID FUTURE KIDNEY INFECTIONS

Maintain Hydration by Drinking Enough Water
One of the best methods to avoid kidney infections is to drink plenty of water. Drinking enough water aids in removing germs from the urinary system before they have a chance to infect the body. Aim for 8 to 10 glasses of water a day, but remember to modify this amount depending on your requirements, activity level, and local environment. Urine that is clear or light in color is a sign of excellent hydration.

Maintain Proper Hygiene

Maintaining proper personal hygiene is crucial to stopping the growth of germs that may lead to kidney diseases. To stop germs from the anal area from entering the urethra, it's crucial for women to wipe after using the toilet from front to back. To lower the danger of bacterial infection, both men and women should wash their genital areas twice a day with mild soap and water, particularly before and after sexual activity.

Frequently and thoroughly urinate

Avoid holding onto pee for long periods of time, as this might lead to an increased risk of urinary tract bacterial development. Every time you urinate, be sure to completely empty your bladder. Urinating helps flush out any germs that may have entered the urethra during sexual activity, which makes it particularly vital afterward. Seek medical attention to rule out any underlying concerns if you often feel the need to pee but only produce little volumes of urine.

Prevent Urinary Tract Irritants

Some products have the potential to aggravate the urinary system and raise the risk of infection. The normal balance of germs in the vaginal region may be upset and the urethra irritated by strong soaps, douches, or feminine hygiene sprays. Choose gentle, fragrance-free products instead. Wearing synthetic undergarments or tight-fitting jeans may also trap moisture and foster the development of germs. Therefore, avoid wearing such items. Instead, choose cotton underwear that is breathable.

Adopt a Kidney-Friendly Diet

Overall renal health is supported by eating a balanced diet high in fruits, vegetables, whole grains, and lean meats. Antioxidant-rich foods like spinach, tomatoes, and berries may help prevent infections and decrease inflammation. Reducing your consumption of processed foods, sugar, and salt may help prevent renal strain and other health problems that can raise your risk of infection. It's crucial to reduce salt intake and stay away from foods rich in oxalates, such as spinach and almonds, for those who have a history of kidney stones.

Boost Your Immune Response

Your first line of protection against infections, especially kidney infections, is a robust immune system. You can strengthen your immune system by eating a balanced diet, exercising frequently, getting adequate sleep, and controlling stress. If your doctor advises it, think about taking a daily multivitamin. Additionally, make sure all of your immunizations are current, especially the ones that guard against bacterial illnesses.

Use medication with caution.

Certain treatments, such as antibiotics and nonsteroidal anti-inflammatory drugs (NSAIDs), may be harsh on the kidneys, particularly if used often or in large quantities. When taking any drug, always adhere to your doctor's recommendations and refrain from self-medicating. Ask your doctor about kidney-safe drugs, especially if you have a history of renal disease or infections.

Handle long-term illnesses

Kidney infections and other kidney-related problems may be made more likely by long-term illnesses such as diabetes and high blood pressure. It's essential to treat these illnesses correctly in order to avoid renal issues. Maintaining blood sugar levels within the intended range may help diabetics' kidneys stay healthy. The key to lessening the burden on the kidneys for those with high blood pressure is to keep it within a healthy range via nutrition, exercise, and medication.

Take into account probiotics.

Probiotics are beneficial bacteria that may lower the risk of infections by supporting a balanced population of microorganisms in the urinary system and stomach. Fermented veggies, kefir, and yogurt are examples of foods that naturally contain probiotics. Probiotic supplements are also an option, but it's advisable to speak with your doctor before beginning any new supplement regimen, particularly if you've had kidney infections in the past.

Use cranberry products with caution. Since cranberry juice may help stop germs from sticking to the bladder wall, cranberry juice and supplements have long been advised for urinary tract health. Although the data is conflicting, some research indicates that cranberry products may help prevent urinary tract infections from recurring, which, if ignored, may result in kidney infections. If you decide to use cranberry products, make sure they are suitable for your situation by speaking with your healthcare provider and choosing pure, unsweetened juice or standardized supplements.

Engage in Safe Sexual Behavior

The risk of infection may rise as germs enter the urinary system during sexual activity. Use condoms with sexual activity, and urinate soon after to lower your risk. To lessen the chance of germs getting into the urethra, women may find it beneficial to clean their vaginal region both before and after intercourse. Your healthcare practitioner may suggest extra preventative measures, including taking a low-dose antibiotic after sexual activity, if recurring illnesses are linked to sexual activity.

Seek Urinary Tract Infection Treatment (UTIs) as Soon as Possible.

Kidney infections can develop very quickly from untreated or poorly managed UTIs. Seek medical attention right away if you have any UTI symptoms, such as burning while urinating, frequent impulses to pee, or cloudy or foul-smelling urine. Antibiotic therapy administered early on may halt the infection from spreading to the kidneys, averting more severe consequences.

Frequent Health Examinations

Monitoring kidney health requires regular check-ups with your healthcare practitioner, particularly if you are at risk for renal disease or have a history of kidney infections. At these appointments, your doctor may run tests to look for any early indications of kidney issues and give tailored guidance on avoiding infections in the future. Regular health monitoring lowers the risk of serious kidney impairment by enabling early management in the event that problems emerge.

Preventive Measures and Hygiene Practices

Daily schedule for personal hygiene

Make personal cleanliness a regular habit to lower your risk of illness. Use water and a light, fragrance-free soap to gently wash the genital region. Steer clear of strong soaps, douches, and feminine sprays since these may upset the bacteria's normal equilibrium. Make sure you wash well, particularly after having sex, to reduce the amount of microorganisms present.

Appropriate Wiping Methods

It's important for women to wipe after using the restroom from front to back. By keeping microorganisms from the anal area from entering the urethra, this procedure lowers the incidence of urinary tract infections (UTIs). Clean toilet paper should be used by both sexes; excessive wiping might irritate surfaces.

Continual personal cleaning

Frequent urination aids in the urinary tract's bacterial removal. Make it a habit to urinate whenever you feel the need, and refrain from holding on to pee for extended periods of time. If you have a history of recurring infections, you may want to think about planning frequent toilet breaks to keep your bladder healthy.

After-Sex Cleaning

Urinating soon after a sexual encounter aids in the removal of any germs that could have entered the urethra during the sexual encounter. Before and after intercourse, both partners should practice proper genital hygiene. Reducing the bacterial burden may be achieved by washing the vaginal region with water before sexual activity.

Fluid intake and hydration

By encouraging regular urine output and eliminating pathogens. Make it a daily goal to consume 8–10 glasses of water. Drink extra water to help the illness heal up faster if you have signs of a urinary tract infection.

Choosing appropriate clothing

Instead of wearing tight clothes that may trap moisture and provide a heated environment for the development of germs, choose breathable cotton underwear. Choose clothing that is loose-fitting and wicks away perspiration while engaging in strenuous activity or in hot conditions. Quickly change out of wet clothes to prevent extended exposure to wetness.

Steer Clear of Irritants

Avoid goods like scented tampons, pads, and feminine hygiene sprays that might irritate the urinary system. These products have the potential to irritate and upset the normal bacterial balance. To reduce irritation, choose unscented or hypoallergenic alternatives.

The Appropriate and Safe Use of Drugs

Follow your doctor's instructions about the use of antibiotics and other drugs, and finish the whole course of therapy. Antibiotic resistance may result from improper or excessive use of antibiotics, which also raises the risk of recurring infections. Before making any adjustments, talk to your healthcare professional about any concerns you may have about a medicine.

Healthy lifestyle choices

To promote kidney and urinary health in general, keep up a healthy lifestyle. Consume less processed food, high-sodium meals, and sugary beverages in favor of a balanced diet full of fruits, vegetables, and whole grains. Regular exercise may improve overall health and reduce stress, which can weaken your immune system.

Regular Medical Exams

Make an appointment for routine health examinations with your physician to keep an eye on the condition of your kidneys and urinary system. Frequent screenings may aid in the early detection of any problems and enable timely treatment. During these appointments, talk to your physician about any symptoms or concerns you may be experiencing to ensure proactive health management.

Teaching Others and Yourself

Learn about kidney infection and urinary tract health prevention strategies. Inform those around you and yourself about proper hygiene habits and the importance of treating infection symptoms as soon as possible. Being informed and conscious of your surroundings might enable you to take charge of your health maintenance.

Avoid using unnecessary catheters.

Employ a urinary catheter properly and dispose of it promptly. If catheter care is not taken appropriately, it might raise the risk of UTIs. To reduce the risk of infection, take care of your catheters according to the instructions provided by your healthcare professional.

Utilizing Probiotics

Probiotics may help maintain a healthy balance of microorganisms in the urinary system, so think about including them in your diet. Probiotics may help maintain general urinary health and can be found in foods like yogurt and kefir as well as supplements. Be sure to speak with your doctor before beginning any new supplement regimen.

Early symptom identification
Be mindful of the early signs of urinary tract infections, which include burning while urinating, frequent desires to go to the bathroom, or murky, bad-smelling urine. Kidney infections are one example of a serious illness that may be avoided by early identification and timely treatment of infections.

PERSONAL HEALTH CHECKUPS' ROLE

Early Health Problem Identification

Frequent medical examinations are essential for the early identification of any health problems, including kidney and urinary tract disorders. Regular examinations and screenings may detect renal dysfunction, infections, and other associated disorders early on, before they worsen. Timely intervention and treatment are made possible by early identification, which may reduce problems and enhance long-term results.

Tracking Kidney Function

Regular check-ups are crucial for monitoring kidney function in those with a history of renal problems or in those who are at risk for kidney disease. Tests for creatinine, blood urea nitrogen (BUN), and glomerular filtration rate (GFR) provide important insights into the kidneys' capacity to remove waste from the blood. Frequent monitoring aids in the early detection of any deterioration in kidney function, enabling proper therapy and halting the development of chronic renal disease.

Evaluating Risk Elements

Checkups provide a chance to evaluate and control risk factors, such as obesity, diabetes, and high blood pressure, that might affect kidney function. In addition to assessing these risk factors, your healthcare professional may provide tailored lifestyle modification recommendations and, if required, write prescriptions for medicines. Proactively addressing these risk factors may lower the likelihood of renal disease and other associated problems.

Assessing the Treatment's Effectiveness

Regular check-ups are essential for assessing how well a patient is responding to therapy for kidney infections or other diseases. During follow-up visits, your healthcare practitioner may evaluate your progress, determine if the therapy is functioning as intended, and make any required modifications. This guarantees that you get the best care possible and lessens the chance of treatment failure or infection recurrence.

Taking care of chronic illnesses

For the proper management of chronic illnesses that might impact kidney function, such as diabetes or hypertension, regular check-ups are essential. Chronic illness care and ongoing monitoring can avoid consequences, such as kidney impairment. Your healthcare practitioner may help you manage chronic diseases by modifying treatment programs, offering support, and offering advice on how to manage symptoms.

Revising Immunization Schedules and Preventive Measures

Updated immunizations and other preventative measures might be discussed during health check-ups. Maintaining current immunizations, such as those for influenza or pneumonia, is critical for the general health of those who are susceptible to illnesses or have compromised immune systems. Advice on additional preventative steps to lower the risk of infections and associated problems may also be given by your healthcare professional.

Handling symptoms and health issues

You may share any symptoms or health issues with your healthcare practitioner at routine check-ups.

These consultations provide an opportunity to discuss any issues you may have about your health, whether they are related to new symptoms, modifications to current problems, or general wellbeing. Maintaining open lines of contact with your supplier guarantees that any problems are looked into and handled properly.

Encouraging preventive healthcare practices

Your healthcare professional may give advice on preventative health measures that promote general well-being during check-ups. Advice on nutrition, exercise, stress reduction, and other lifestyle choices that support kidney health and general health may fall under this category. Preventive care encourages a better lifestyle and lowers the chance of health issues.

Monitoring Health Patterns Through Time

Frequent examinations allow us to monitor changes in health over time. Through the process of cross-referencing current health information with earlier data, your healthcare professional may see trends, track modifications, and evaluate how any issues are developing. Making choices about treatment and preventative measures is made easier with this long-term view in mind.

Improving patient involvement and education

Checkups provide a chance for patient involvement and education. In addition to discussing the implications of your current health state and offering advice for preserving or enhancing your health, your healthcare professional may also interpret test findings. You may actively manage your health and make lifestyle habits that promote kidney health when you are knowledgeable and involved in your healthcare decisions.

Creating a Solid Patient-Provider Bond

Establishing a solid and trustworthy rapport with your healthcare practitioner is facilitated by regular check-ups. This continuous interaction guarantees that your healthcare professional is knowledgeable about your medical background, is aware of your requirements, and is able to provide individualized treatment. Stronger relationships between patients and providers facilitate greater communication, raise the standard of treatment, and promote improved health outcomes.

CONCLUSION: EMPOWERING YOUR KIDNEY HEALTH JOURNEY

Taking control of your kidney health requires a proactive, all-encompassing strategy that incorporates routine care, prevention, and awareness. You may support your kidneys' optimum function and avoid issues by making educated choices based on your knowledge of the critical role that kidneys play in sustaining overall health.

Preventative Action

Prevention is the foundation for kidney health. Renal infections and other kidney-related problems may be considerably decreased by adopting a lifestyle that includes enough water, good cleanliness, a balanced diet, and frequent exercise. Implementing these routines may foster renal function and reduce the risk of developing health   issues.

Early identification and consistent monitoring

Regular check-ups are crucial for kidney disease early diagnosis and treatment. Regular tests make it possible to identify any problems early on, which facilitates appropriate intervention and treatment. Regular consultations for risk assessment and kidney function monitoring assist in successfully managing chronic illnesses, stopping their development, and preserving general health.

Combining Medical and Natural Methods

Supplementing traditional medical care with

homeopathic medicines may speed healing and promote renal function. You may support a holistic approach to health and supplement medical therapies with natural methods, including dietary changes, stress reduction, and herbal supplements, while working with medical specialists.

Developing Your Own Knowledge to Empower You

Knowledge is a great way to take care of your kidneys. You are more equipped to make decisions and take proactive action if you are aware of the symptoms, risk factors, and preventative actions. Being informed about your health and available treatments enables you to take an active role in your care and work well with your healthcare practitioner.

Creating a Supportive Healthcare Partnership

A positive working relationship with your physician is essential to effectively managing the health of your kidneys. Enhancing your care experience and improving health outcomes is possible via a supportive relationship that is fostered by regular communication, adherence to treatment plans, and involvement in decision-making.

Dedication to Prolonged Well-being

Kidney health requires constant attention and maintenance. You may guarantee long-term health and well-being by consistently putting preventative tactics into practice, following treatment regimens, and going in for frequent checkups. With a dedicated attitude, embrace this path, understanding that every action you take will lead to a better future.

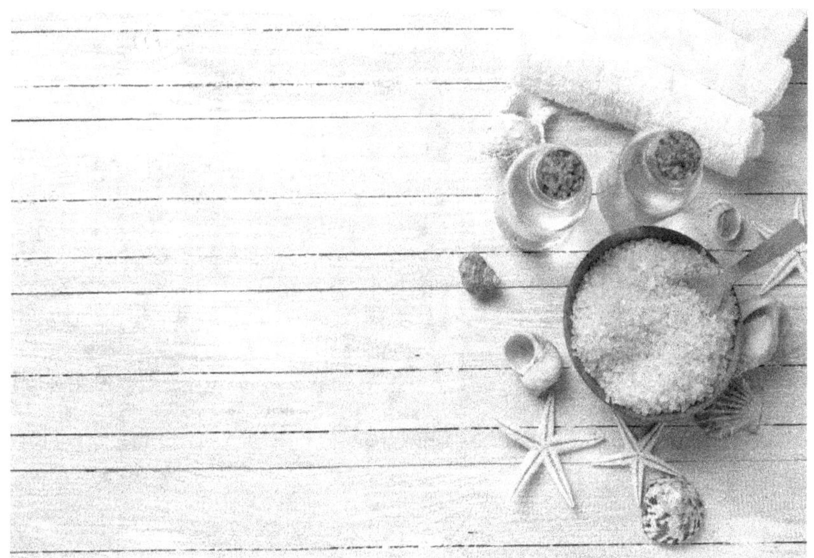

Walnut

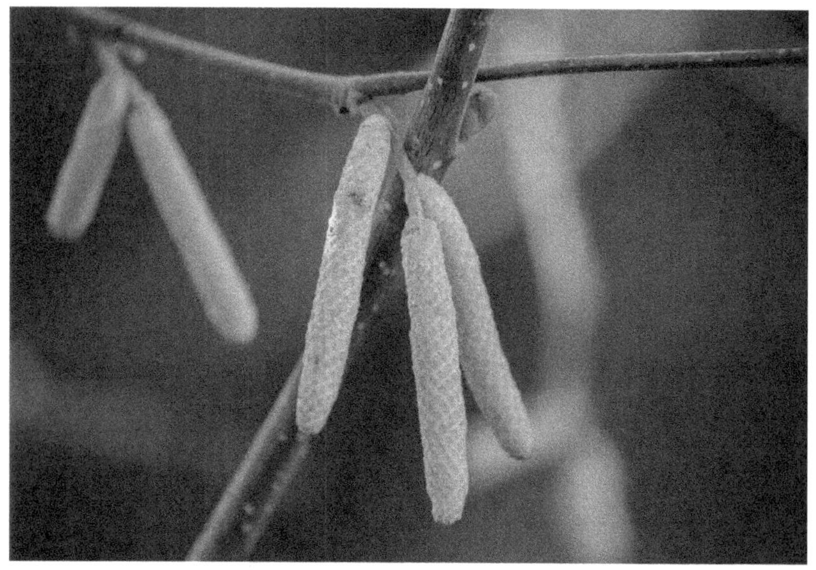

SUMMARY OF KEY TAKEAWAYS

Prioritize Prevention: Lowering the risk of kidney infections and enhancing general kidney health require adopting preventive measures, such as drinking enough water, practicing excellent hygiene, and eating a diet that is easy on the kidneys.

I agree to conduct regular health exams. Ups: Make time for regular physical examinations to track kidney function, identify any problems early, and successfully manage risk factors. To avoid major issues and provide preventive treatment, regular screenings are necessary.

Incorporate natural solutions. Use natural therapies, such as stress reduction techniques and dietary modifications, in addition to conventional therapy, as directed by your healthcare professional. This all-encompassing strategy may promote long-term kidney health and speed up recovery.

Educate Yourself: Keep up to date on kidney health, possible problem signs, and preventative measures. Having knowledge gives you the ability to actively control your health and make wise choices.

Create a Solid Healthcare Partnership: Encourage cooperation between you and your healthcare provider. Improved health outcomes may be attained via active participation in your care, strict adherence to treatment regimens, and open communication.

Adopt a holistic lifestyle: include stress management, regular exercise, a balanced diet, and abstaining from dangerous drugs in your daily routine. These routines promote general wellbeing and renal health.

Put Long-Term Health First: Make a commitment to preserving kidney health via continuous screening, proactive well-being, and preventative actions. Every action you take now will benefit a healthy tomorrow.

Motivating the Integration of Healthful Habits

Developing healthy behaviors as part of your

everyday routine will empower you to control your kidney health. You can greatly improve the health of your kidneys and your overall quality of life by making educated lifestyle decisions, scheduling regular checkups, and prioritizing preventative care. Adopt a comprehensive strategy that consists of a healthy diet, enough water, frequent exercise, and efficient stress reduction. Your commitment to these beneficial behaviors promotes long-term health and vigor in addition to renal function.

A better, more satisfying existence is only one step away from every constructive adjustment you make.

BOOK REVIEW

Title: Kidney Supporting Recovery at Home: Natural Remedies and Lifestyle Changes for Kidney Health

Author: Dr. Esther J. Ramage

Overall Rating:

☆☆☆☆☆ (Please rate the book on a scale of 1 to 5 stars)

Content Quality: Relevance:

How relevant and useful was the content for your needs?

Rating: ☆☆☆☆☆

Clarity: Was the information clearly presented and easy to understand?

Rating: ☆ ☆ ☆ ☆ ☆

Depth: Did the book cover the topic comprehensively?

Rating: ☆ ☆ ☆ ☆ ☆

Practical Application: Usability: Were the natural remedies and lifestyle changes easy to implement?

Rating: ☆ ☆ ☆ ☆ ☆

Impact: Did you notice any improvements in your health or well-being after applying the book's suggestions?

Rating: ☆ ☆ ☆ ☆ ☆

Writing Style: Engagement: Was the writing engaging and did it maintain your interest throughout?

Rating: ☆ ☆ ☆ ☆ ☆

Tone: Was the tone of the book approachable and reader-friendly?

Rating: ★ ★ ★ ★ ☆

Design and Layout:

Visual Appeal: How appealing was the book's layout and design?

Rating: ☆ ☆ ☆ ☆ ☆

Ease of Navigation: Was it easy to navigate through the chapters and sections?

Rating: ☆ ☆ ☆ ☆ ☆

Specific Feedback:

Favorite Sections: Which sections or chapters did you find most helpful or interesting? Why?

Suggestions for Improvement: Is there anything you think could be improved in the book? Please provide details.

Personal Experience:

Biggest Takeaway: What was your biggest takeaway or learning from this book?

Recommendation: Would you recommend this book to others? Why or why not?

Additional Comments: Please feel free to add any additional thoughts or comments about the book.

Conclusion:

Thank you for sharing your review! Your feedback is greatly appreciated and will help guide others in their reading choices.